This publication is a collection of resources for consumers on the topics of weight management and obesity. The resources on this list are in a variety of information formats: articles, pamphlets, books, and full-text materials on the World Wide Web.

This list was developed to provide reliable nutrition information about weight loss, weight management, and obesity, and is not intended to provide specific medical advice. The Food and Nutrition Information Center (FNIC) urges individuals to consult with a qualified physician or Registered Dietitian (RD) for answers to specific questions.

Materials included in this list may also be available to borrow from the National Agricultural Library (NAL). Lending and copy service information is provided at the end of this document. If you are not eligible for direct borrowing privileges, check with your local library on how to borrow through interlibrary loan. Materials cannot be purchased from NAL. Contact information is provided if you wish to purchase any materials on this list.

Each item has been placed in one or more of the following sections, and may be organized by resource type (e.g., book, brochure, Web site):

A. Defining Overweight and Obesity
    1. Definitions
    2. Trends, Statistics, and Costs
B. Health Effects of Overweight and Obesity
C. Resources for Weight Management and Obesity Prevention
    1. General Resources
    2. Interactive Weight Management Tools
    3. Evaluating Popular Diets and Weight Loss Methods
    4. Supervised Approaches to Weight Loss
D. Weight Management Resources for Children and Adolescents

A. Defining Overweight and Obesity

1. Definitions

BMI – Body Mass Index
Department of Health and Human Services (DHHS), Centers for Disease Control and Prevention (CDC), National Center for Chronic Disease Prevention and Health Promotion
Web site: http://www.cdc.gov/nccdphp/dnpa/bmi/index.htm
Description: Provides a definition for BMI as well as separate BMI calculators for adults and for children and teens. Additional nutrition, weight and health resources are also available.

Defining Overweight and Obesity
DHHS, CDC, National Center for Chronic Disease Prevention and Health Promotion
Web site: http://www.cdc.gov/nccdphp/dnpa/obesity/defining.htm
Description: Discusses obesity and obesity measures while detailing dangers and risks. Defines overweight and obesity for adults, children and teens.

Obesity Information
American Heart Association
Web site:
http://www.heart.org/HEARTORG/GettingHealthy/WeightManagement/Obesity/Obesity-Information_UCM_307908_Article.jsp
Description: Provides definitions for obesity and links to information on achieving a healthy weight.

Weight-control Information Network (WIN)
DHHS, National Institutes of Health (NIH), National Institute for Diabetes and Digestive and Kidney Diseases
Web site: http://win.niddk.nih.gov/index.htm
Description: Provides the general public, health professionals, the media, and Congress with up-to-date, science-based information on weight control, obesity, physical activity, and related nutritional issues.
Ordering Information:
The Weight-control Information Network
1 WIN Way
Bethesda, MD 20892-3665
Phone: 1-877-946-4627   Fax: 202-828-1028
Publications Order Form: http://win.niddk.nih.gov/order/orderpub.htm
Email: win@info.niddk.nih.gov

> **Obesity, Physical Activity, and Weight Control Glossary**
> **Full text:** http://win.niddk.nih.gov/publications/glossary.htm
> **Description:** Defines words that are often used when people talk or write about obesity, physical activity, and weight control.

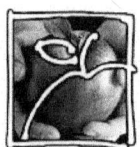

Understanding Adult Obesity
Full text: http://win.niddk.nih.gov/publications/understanding.htm
Description: Provides definitions of overweight and obesity including BMI and body fat distribution. Also discusses possible causes, health consequences, prevention and treatment of overweight and obesity.

Weight and Waist Measurement: Tools for Adults
Full text: http://win.niddk.nih.gov/publications/tools.htm
Description: Explains how to measure BMI and waist circumference, and what these measures mean for your health.

What are Overweight and Obesity?
DHHS, NIH, National Heart Lung and Blood Institute
Web site: http://www.nhlbi.nih.gov/health/dci/Diseases/obe/obe_whatare.html
Description: Defines overweight and obesity, and identifies possible causes of each, who is at risk, treatment, prevention, and more.

2. Trends, Statistics, and Costs

Overweight and Obesity: Causes and Consequences
DHHS, CDC, National Center for Chronic Disease Prevention and Health Promotion
Web site: http://www.cdc.gov/obesity/adult/causes/index.html
Description: Discusses variety of factors that play a role in obesity, including behavior, environment and genetic factors. Also includes information on the health and economic consequences of overweight and obesity.

Overweight and Obesity: Data and Statistics
DHHS, CDC, National Center for Chronic Disease Prevention and Health Promotion
Web site: http://www.cdc.gov/obesity/data/index.html
Description: Provides overweight and obesity trends among adults and among children and adolescents, as well as related resources.

Statistics Related to Overweight and Obesity
NIDDK, Weight-control Information Network
Web site: http://win.niddk.nih.gov/statistics/
Description: Provides statistics related to the prevalence, economic costs, and health related risks of overweight and obesity.

U.S. Obesity Trends
DHHS, CDC, National Center for Chronic Disease Prevention and Health Promotion
Web site: http://www.cdc.gov/obesity/data/trends.html
Description: Shows the increase in U.S. obesity rates by state and by year in a series of Power Point slides. Slides provide a visual image of the increased prevalence of obesity across each of the states.

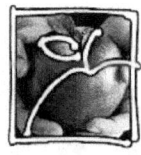

B. Health Effects of Overweight and Obesity

The Health Effects of Overweight and Obesity
DHHS, CDC, National Center for Chronic Disease Prevention and Health Promotion
Web site: http://www.cdc.gov/healthyweight/effects/index.html
Description: Lists health conditions for which overweight and obesity lead to higher risk.

Obesity Fact Sheets
The Obesity Society
Web site: http://www.obesity.org/resources-for/fact-sheets.htm
Description: Provides information regarding the health impacts of obesity. Specific fact sheets on health-related outcomes include:
- What is Obesity?: http://www.obesity.org/resources-for/what-is-obesity.htm
- Obesity and Diabetes: http://www.obesity.org/resources-for/your-weight-and-diabetes.htm
- Obesity and Cancer: http://www.obesity.org/resources-for/cancer-and-obesity.htm
- Childhood Overweight: http://www.obesity.org/resources-for/childhood-overweight.htm
- Obesity, Bias and Stigmatization: http://www.obesity.org/resources-for/obesity-bias-and-stigmatization.htm

Obesity – Stroke Connection
American Heart Association
Web site:
http://www.heart.org/HEARTORG/GettingHealthy/WeightManagement/Obesity/Obesity---Stroke-Connection_UCM_311771_Article.jsp
Description: Discusses the connection between obesity and stroke.

Overweight and Obesity: Health Consequences
DHHS, Office of the Surgeon General
Web site: http://www.surgeongeneral.gov/library/calls/obesity/fact_consequences.html
Description: Reviews potential health consequences, or conditions, resulting from overweight and obesity, and provides benefits of weight loss.

Weight-control Information Network
DHHS, NIH, National Institute for Diabetes and Digestive and Kidney Diseases
Web site: http://win.niddk.nih.gov/index.htm
Description: Provides the general public, health professionals, the media, and Congress with up-to-date, science-based information on weight control, obesity, physical activity, and related nutritional issues.
Ordering Information:
The Weight-control Information Network
1 WIN Way
Bethesda, MD 20892-3665

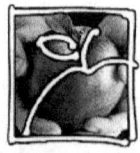

Phone: 1-877-946-4627   Fax: 202-828-1028
Publications Order Form: http://win.niddk.nih.gov/order/orderpub.htm
Email: win@info.niddk.nih.gov

Do You Know the Health Risks of Being Overweight?
Full text: http://win.niddk.nih.gov/publications/health_risks.htm
Description: Provides information about the health risks which may be increased by overweight and obesity.

Weight Cycling
Full text: http://www.niddk.nih.gov/health/nutrit/pubs/wcycling.htm
Description: Discusses the myths and realities of repeated weight loss and regain.

What Are the Health Risks of Overweight and Obesity?
DHHS, NIH, National Heart, Lung and Blood Institute
Web site: http://www.nhlbi.nih.gov/health/health-topics/topics/obe/risks.html
Description: Reviews overweight and obesity-related health problems in adults.

C. Resources for Weight Management and Obesity Prevention

1. General Resources

Books

American Dietetic Association Complete Food and Nutrition Guide, 4th Edition
Roberta Larson Duyff, MS, RD, FADA, CFCS
Hoboken, NJ: John Wiley & Sons, Inc., 2012, 720 pp.
ISBN: 978-0470912072
NAL Call Number: RA784 .D89 2012
Description: Addresses healthy eating guidelines and strategies for adults, teens, and children. Includes chapters on food intolerance and allergies, vegetarian eating, athletics and nutrition, and dietary supplements. Discusses how to spot health quackery and when to seek the advice of a nutrition professional.

Bite It & Write It!
Stacie Castle, MS, RD, CDN, Robyn A. Cotler, MS, RD, CDN, Marni Schefter, RD, CDN, Shana Shapiro, MS, RD, CDN, CDE
New York: Square One Publishers, 2011, 192 pp.
ISBN: 0757003435
Description: Provides ten weekly health goals, which can be personalized, with tips to help reach them. This book also serves as a nutrition journal to help you keep track of your intake. Also includes calorie guides for common foods and chain restaurant foods.

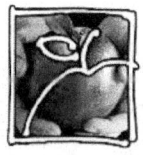

The Calorie Counter, 5th Edition

Karen Nolan, PhD and Jo-Ann Heslin, MA, RD
New York: Pocket Books, 2010, 704 pp.
ISBN: 1-4165-6667-0
Description: Provides calorie counts for more than 20,000 foods, including over 800 take-out foods and 100 restaurant chains. Introductory text offers information on energy (calorie) needs and portion control.

Eat Out, Eat Right: The Guide to Healthier Restaurant Eating, 3rd Edition

Hope Warshaw, MMSc, RD, CDE
Chicago, IL: Surrey Books, 2008, 284 pp.
ISBN: 1572840927
Description: Provides an overview of restaurant eating habits and introduces skills and strategies that can be used at any restaurant to make healthier choices. Includes nutrition information for a variety of restaurant foods and cuisines, and offers tips for decoding "menu lingo."

Eat Right When Time is Tight: 150 Slim-Down Strategies and No-Cook Food Fixes

Patricia Bannan, MS, RD
Bedford, IN: NorlightsPress.Com, 2010, 206 pp.
ISBN: 1935254294
Description: Written specifically for women, offers research and ten master strategies, in addition to mini-strategies and meal suggestions, to "eat right when time is tight." Includes practical meals and snacks.

The Instinct Diet: Use Your Five Food Instincts to Lose Weight and Keep It Off

Susan Roberts, PhD and Betty Kelly Sargent
New York: Workman Publishing, 2008, 338 pp.
ISBN: 0761150196
Description: Defines five basic "food instincts" (hunger, availability, calorie density, familiarity and variety) and teaches readers to work with them rather than against them to manage what, how, when and how much they eat over the course of an 8-week program. Recipes and appendices, including a savvy supermarket shopper directory and sample food diary, are included.

Intuitive Eating: A Revolutionary Program That Works, 3rd Edition

Evelyn Tribole, MS, RD, and Elyse Resch, MS, RD, FADA
New York: St. Martin's Press, 2012, 344 pp.
ISBN: 1250004047
Description: Encourages thoughtful eating behaviors, such as eating when hungry, challenging the traditional "dieting" mentality, and respecting your body, to reach weight loss or maintenance goals.

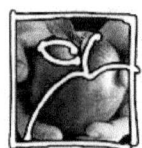

The Mayo Clinic Diet: Eat Well, Enjoy Life, Lose Weight
Mayo Foundation for Medical Education and Research
Intercourse, PA: Good Books, 2010, 254 pp.
ISBN: 1561486760
Description: Offers a two part plan (Part One: Lose It, Part Two: Live It) for individuals to achieve long-term, sustainable weight loss through behavior changes; provides tips for meal planning and eating out.

Mindless Eating: Why We Eat More Than We Think
Brian Wansink, PhD
New York: Bantam Books, 2010, 304 pp.
ISBN: 978-0-345-52688-5
Description: Discusses why, how much, and what people are eating—often without realizing it. Provides "reengineering strategies" to help curb mindless eating behaviors. Appendices compare popular diet plans and give tips for "defusing your diet danger zones."

The Most Complete Food Counter, 3rd Edition
Karen J. Nolan, PhD and Jo-Ann Heslin, MA, RD
New York: Gallery Books, 2013, 965 pp.
ISBN: 978-1-4516-2164-8
Description: Provides nutrient values, including calories, fat, cholesterol, protein, carbohydrates, fiber, sodium, and more for over 21,000 foods. Introductory text offers information on how to adequately eat or limit the above nutrients, and provides an A-Z "dictionary" of food and nutrition terms and concepts.

The Ultimate Volumetrics Diet: Smart, Simple, Science-Based Strategies for Losing Weight and Keeping It Off
Barbara Rolls, PhD with Mindy Hermann, RD
New York: HarperCollins, 2012, 416 pp.
ISBN: 978-0062060648
Description: Shows how to select foods that provide satisfying portions while still allowing people to feel full on fewer calories. Includes recipes, budget and time-saving tips, charts, and photos.

Brochures, Booklets, and Tools

Aim for a Healthy Weight
DHHS, NIH, National Heart, Lung and Blood Institute
NHLBI Publication No. 05-5213
Web site: http://www.nhlbi.nih.gov/health/public/heart/obesity/aim_hwt.htm
Description: Contains practical, easy-to-use information for losing and maintaining weight, including tips on healthy eating and physical activity, setting weight loss goals, and rewarding success. Also includes portion and serving size information, sample reduced calorie menus, tips on dining out, a sample walking program, and a weekly food and activity diary.

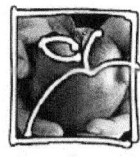

Ordering Information:
NHLBI Health Information Center
P.O. Box 30105
Bethesda, MD 20824-0105
Phone: 301-592-8573   Fax: 240-629-3246
Email: NHLBIinfo@nhlbi.nih.gov
Web site: http://www.nhlbi.nih.gov/index.htm

Drawing the Line on Calories, Carbs, and Fats
Roberta Schwartz Wennik, MS, RD
Web site: http://www.advantagediets.com/drawingtheline.htm
Description: Allows users to track food intake and exercise by connecting a series of dots ("drawing the line"), rather than writing down all foods eaten. Available for purchase in hard copy, downloadable eBook, and DVD from the Web site.
Online Ordering: http://www.advantagediets.com/buynow.htm

Let's Eat for the Health of It
U.S. Department of Agriculture; U.S. Department of Health and Human Services
Web site: http://www.cnpp.usda.gov/publications/myplate/dg2010brochure.pdf (PDF|968 KB)
Description: Consumer brochure that provides tips for healthful eating and being active based on recommendations from the *2010 Dietary Guidelines for Americans* and MyPlate.

Watch Your Weight!/¡Cuide Su Peso!
DHHS, NIH, National Heart, Lung and Blood Institute
NHLBI Publication No. 96-4047
Full text: http://www.nhlbi.nih.gov/health/public/heart/other/sp_wt.pdf (PDF|412 KB)
Description: Written especially for Latino families, these bilingual booklets (English and Spanish) describe healthy dietary changes people can make to reduce their risk of having a heart attack or stroke.

Weight-control Information Network
DHHS, NIH, National Institute for Diabetes and Digestive and Kidney Diseases
Web site: http://win.niddk.nih.gov/index.htm
Description: Provides the general public, health professionals, the media, and Congress with up-to-date, science-based information on weight control, obesity, physical activity, and related nutritional issues.
Ordering Information:
The Weight-control Information Network
1 WIN Way
Bethesda, MD 20892-3665
Phone: 1-877-946-4627   Fax: 202-828-1028
Publications Order Form: http://win.niddk.nih.gov/order/orderpub.htm
Email: win@info.niddk.nih.gov

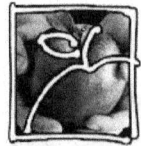

Active at Any Size
Full text: http://win.niddk.nih.gov/publications/active.htm
Description: Encourages physical activity for individuals of any size. Suggested physical activities and safety tips are provided, as well as resources to get started.

Better Health and You: Tips for Adults
Full text: http://win.niddk.nih.gov/publications/better_health.htm
Description: Provides tips for eating right and being active to help individuals reach or maintain a healthy weight.

Cómo Alimentarse y Mantenerse Activo Durante Toda La Vida (Healthy Eating & Physical Activity Across Your Lifespan)
Full text: http://win.niddk.nih.gov/publications/para_adultos.htm
Description: Discusses how eating well and physical activity contribute to healthy living.

Improving Your Health: Tips for African American Men and Women
Full text: http://win.niddk.nih.gov/publications/improving.htm
Description: Provides tips for making changes to physical activity and eating habits that can improve health.

Just Enough For You: About Food Portions
Full text: http://win.niddk.nih.gov/publications/just_enough.htm
Description: Discusses the difference between portions and serving sizes, and shows how to identify serving sizes by comparing them to everyday objects.

Physical Activity and Weight Control
Full text: http://win.niddk.nih.gov/publications/physical.htm
Description: Discusses the importance of physical activity and provides tips for a safe physical activity program.

Sisters Together: Move More, Eat Better
- Energize Yourself & Your Family
  Full text: http://win.niddk.nih.gov/publications/energize.htm
- Fit and Fabulous as You Mature
  Full text: http://win.niddk.nih.gov/publications/mature.htm

Description: Sisters Together: Move More, Eat Better is a national media-based program designed to encourage African American women 18 and over to maintain a healthy weight by becoming more physically active and eating healthier foods.

Weight Loss for Life
Full text: http://win.niddk.nih.gov/publications/for_life.htm
Description: Gives an overview of overweight, the types of programs available for weight loss, portion size, and other weight control strategies.

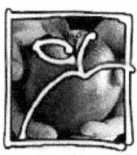

Web Sites

Aim for a Healthy Weight
DHHS, NIH, National Heart, Lung and Blood Institute
Web site: http://www.nhlbi.nih.gov/health/public/heart/obesity/lose_wt/
Description: Summarizes key recommendations for weight loss, and allows users to assess their risk factors related to overweight or obesity. Also provides interactive tools and links to physical activity and behavior change guides, shopping tips, recipes, sample menus and a daily food diary to help people get started.

Back to Basics for Healthy Weight Loss
Academy of Nutrition and Dietetics
Web site: http://www.eatright.org/public/content.aspx?id=6847
Description: Details three basic steps for weight loss success.

Belly Fat in Men: Why Weight Loss Matters
MayoClinic.com, Mayo Foundation for Medical Education and Research
Web site: http://www.mayoclinic.com/health/belly-fat/MC00054
Description: Discusses health risks linked to excess abdominal fat in men.

Belly Fat in Women: Taking – and Keeping – It Off
MayoClinic.com, Mayo Foundation for Medical Education and Research
Web site: http://www.mayoclinic.com/health/belly-fat/WO00128
Description: Examines the risks of abdominal obesity in women, and provides lifestyle tips and targeted abdominal exercises to help flatten the belly and tone the abdominal muscles.

ChooseMyPlate.gov
U.S. Department of Agriculture (USDA), Center for Nutrition Policy and Promotion
Web site: http://www.choosemyplate.gov/
Spanish: http://www.choosemyplate.gov/en-espanol.html
Description: MyPlate incorporates recommendations from the *Dietary Guidelines for Americans, 2010* and offers personalized eating plans, interactive tools to help users plan food choices, and advice on how to balance food and physical activity. See related interactive tools in next section.

Energy Density and Weight Loss: Feel Full on Fewer Calories
MayoClinic.com, Mayo Foundation for Medical Education and Research
Web site: http://www.mayoclinic.com/health/weight-loss/NU00195
Description: Explains the concept of energy density and provides tips for choosing foods that can help people feel full on fewer calories.

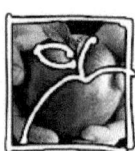

How Can I Manage My Weight
American Heart Association
Web site: http://www.heart.org/HEARTORG/GettingHealthy/How-Can-I-Manage-My-Weight_UCM_308997_Article.jsp
Description: Printable information sheet provides advice on how to reach and maintain a healthy weight.

Lose Weight the Healthy Way
American Institute for Cancer Research
Web site: http://www.aicr.org/site/PageServer?pagename=reduce_weight_healthy_way
Description: Provides a three-step approach to losing weight. Also includes a serving size finder to help control portion sizes.

Losing Weight
American Heart Association
Web site:
http://www.heart.org/HEARTORG/GettingHealthy/WeightManagement/LosingWeight/Losing-Weight_UCM_307904_Article.jsp
Description: Provides links to information reducing calories taken in and increasing calories expended, and links to related resources on goals for healthy eating and losing weight, the *No-Fad Diet*, recognizing roadblocks and keeping weight off.

Menopause Weight Gain: Stop the Middle Age Spread
Mayo Clinic.com, Mayo Foundation for Medical Education and Research
Web site: http://www.mayoclinic.com/invoke.cfm?id=HQ01076&printpage=true
Description: Describes physical changes that occur during menopause and ways to maintain a healthy weight and a realistic acceptance of inevitable body changes.

The New American Plate
American Institute for Cancer Research
Web site: http://www.aicr.org/new-american-plate
Description: Gives a graphic representation of a healthy portion and plate of food, and invites comparison to people's current proportion of foods and portion sizes on their own plates. Sample menus and recipes are also included.
Publications Ordering: http://www.aicr.org/publications

Nutrition.gov
USDA, National Agricultural Library
Web site: http://www.nutrition.gov
Description: Serves as a gateway to reliable information on nutrition, healthy eating, and physical activity for consumers in the effort to reduce obesity and other food-related diseases. Offers an online article, "Interested in Losing Weight?", that reviews resources and hints for getting started; article is available at http://www.nutrition.gov/losingweight

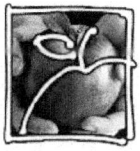

Overweight and Obesity: What You Can Do
DHHS, Office of the Surgeon General
Web site: http://www.surgeongeneral.gov/library/calls/obesity/fact_whatcanyoudo.html
Description: Discusses physical activity approaches (and benefits) to attain or maintain a healthy weight.

Overweight, Obesity and Weight Loss
DHHS, National Women's Health Information Center
Web site: http://www.womenshealth.gov/publications/our-publications/fact-sheet/overweight-weight-loss.html
Description: Addresses health effects of being overweight or obese and gives tips for improving diet and increasing physical activity. Also discusses surgical options for weight loss and how to keep children healthy.

Shape Up!
Shape Up America! Healthy Weight for Life
Web site: http://www.shapeup.org
Description: Aims to raise obesity awareness and provide information for healthy weight management. Provides links to allow users to assess their activity level, flexibility, and endurance, as well as links to other topic areas including activity calculators, "Cyberkitchen" and "10,000 Steps."

Tips for Healthy Eating On the Go or At Home
DHHS, NIH, National Heart, Lung and Blood Institute
Web site: http://www.nhlbi.nih.gov/health/public/heart/obesity/lose_wt/ob_tips.htm
Description: Provides links to various tip sheets including:
    Eating Healthy Starts With Healthy Food Shopping:
    http://www.nhlbi.nih.gov/health/public/heart/obesity/lose_wt/shop.htm
    Eating Healthy When Dining Out:
    http://www.nhlbi.nih.gov/health/public/heart/obesity/lose_wt/dine_out.htm
    Eating Healthy With Ethnic Food:
    http://www.nhlbi.nih.gov/health/public/heart/obesity/lose_wt/eth_dine.htm

What You Should Know Before You Start a Weight Loss Plan
American Academy of Family Physicians
Web site: http://familydoctor.org/online/famdocen/home/healthy/food/improve/788.html
Spanish: http://familydoctor.org/online/famdoces/home/healthy/food/improve/788.html
Description: Discusses the importance of consulting with a doctor before starting a weight loss plan, and provides tips on getting active.

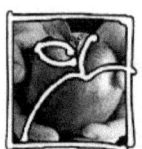

2. Interactive Weight Management Tools

America On the Move
America On the Move Foundation
Web site: https://aom3.americaonthemove.org/
Description: Allows users to keep track of their physical activity (steps) and dietary progress.

BMI – Body Mass Index Calculator
DHHS, CDC, National Center for Chronic Disease Prevention and Health Promotion
Web site: http://www.cdc.gov/nccdphp/dnpa/bmi/index.htm
Description: Calculates body mass index (BMI) for adults, children and teens in both English and Metric measurements.

Cyberkitchen
Shape Up America!
Web site: http://www.shapeup.org/kitchen/kitchen_0.html
Description: Shows how to balance food intake with physical activity. Also provides information on how to achieve and maintain a healthy weight through interactive assessment, meal planning, and recipes.

Healthy Body Calculator
Ask the Dietitian - Joanne Larsen, MS, RD, LD
Web site: http://www.dietitian.com/calcbody.php
Description: Calculates body mass index (BMI), and provides information on nutrient composition, body shape, and corresponding disease risk. This Web site also gives personalized suggested activities for weight loss.

HealthyDiningFinder.com
Healthy Dining
Web site: http://www.healthydiningfinder.com
Description: Searches for healthier meals at restaurants ranging from fast food to fine dining. Corresponding nutrition information such as calories, fat, and sodium is also provided.

How Active Are You? Calorie Calculator
Center for Science in the Public Interest
Web site: http://www.cspinet.org/nah/09_03/calorie_calc.html
Description: Determines a targeted calorie intake determined by a person's gender, age, height, weight and activity level.

Interactive Menu Planner
DHHS, NIH, NHLBI, Obesity Education Initiative
Web site: http://hp2010.nhlbihin.net/menuplanner/menu.cgi
Description: Guides daily food and meal choices based on a person's daily calorie needs.

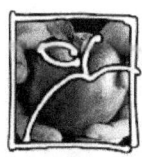

Make Your Calories Count: Use the Nutrition Facts Label for Healthy Weight Management
Food and Drug Administration (FDA), Center for Food Safety and Applied Nutrition
Web site: http://www.fda.gov/Food/ResourcesForYou/Consumers/NFLPM/ucm275438.htm
Description: Interactive learning program that provides users with information to help plan a healthful diet while managing calorie intake.

MyPlate – SuperTracker and Other Tools
USDA, Center for Nutrition Policy and Promotion
Web site: http://www.choosemyplate.gov/supertracker-tools.html
Description: Links to various interactive tools and resources to help users plan, analyze, and track food choices and physical activity. Calorie and fats charts, a BMI calculator, and daily food plans are also included. See direct link to the SuperTracker Web site:
* **SuperTracker:** https://www.supertracker.usda.gov/
  Allows users to compare food choices to recommendations and nutrient needs, assess personal physical activity, and set a personal calorie goal.

Nutriinfo Health eTools
Nutriinfo.com, Minu Interactive, Inc.
Web site: http://www.nutriinfo.com/etools/etools.jsp
Description: Calculates body mass index, waist-to-hip ratio, daily caloric needs, calories burned during exercise, and find local health professionals. Each tool provides information about health status and weight loss goals. eTools are free to download.

Portion Distortion
DHHS, NIH, National Heart, Lung and Blood Institute
Web site: http://hp2010.nhlbihin.net/portion/
Description: Interactive Web site with two quizzes to compare portion sizes now and 20 years ago.

USDA National Nutrient Database for Standard Reference
USDA, Agricultural Research Service, Nutrient Data Laboratory
Web site: http://ndb.nal.usda.gov/
Description: Provides detailed nutrient analysis for over 8,000 foods.

3. Evaluating Popular Diets and Weight Loss Methods

Brochures, Booklets, and Tools

Weight-control Information Network
DHHS, NIH, National Institute for Diabetes and Digestive and Kidney Diseases
Web site: http://win.niddk.nih.gov/index.htm
Description: Provides the general public, health professionals, the media, and Congress with up-to-date, science-based information on weight control, obesity, physical activity, and related nutritional issues.

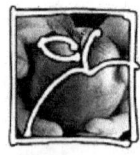

Ordering Information:
The Weight-control Information Network
1 WIN Way
Bethesda, MD 20892-3665
Phone: 1-877-946-4627
Fax: 202-828-1028
Publications Order Form: http://win.niddk.nih.gov/order/orderpub.htm
Email: win@info.niddk.nih.gov

Choosing a Safe and Successful Weight-loss Program
Full text: http://win.niddk.nih.gov/publications/choosing.htm
Description: Provides guidance about speaking to your health care professional about weight loss and gathering the best information before choosing a program.

Weight Cycling
Full text: http://win.niddk.nih.gov/publications/cycling.htm
Description: Discusses the myths and realities of repeated weight loss and regain.

Weight-loss and Nutrition Myths: How Much Do You Really Know?
Full text: http://www.niddk.nih.gov/health/nutrit/pubs/myths/index.htm
Description: Provides information about the myths and realities of weight loss in an easy to follow question and answer format.

Web Sites

Ask the Dietitian: Nutrition Information on the Internet
Cleveland Clinic Heart and Vascular Institute
Web site: http://my.clevelandclinic.org/heart/prevention/askdietician/ask7_01.aspx
Description: Provides strategies for deciphering between a science-based Web site and a less reliable—or even fraudulent—one.

Consumer Diet and Lifestyle Book Reviews
Academy of Nutrition and Dietetics
Web site: http://www.eatright.org/Media/content.aspx?id=264
Description: Provides links to brief reviews of popular diet books by Academy of Nutrition and Dietetics spokespeople.

Evaluating Weight Control Programs
USDA, National Agricultural Library (NAL), Food and Nutrition Information Center
Web site: http://fnic.nal.usda.gov/weight-and-obesity/evaluating-weight-control-programs
Description: Links to a variety of articles, brochures, and publications to help consumers decipher weight and diet claims.

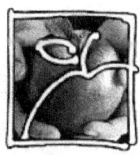

High-Protein Diets

American Heart Association

Web site: http://www.heart.org/HEARTORG/GettingHealthy/NutritionCenter/High-Protein-Diets_UCM_305989_Article.jsp

Description: Background information and a recommendation against high-protein diets from the American Heart Association.

Quick-Weight-Loss or Fad Diets

American Heart Association

Web site: http://www.heart.org/HEARTORG/GettingHealthy/NutritionCenter/Quick-Weight-Loss-or-Fad-Diets_UCM_305970_Article.jsp

Description: Overviews ways to spot fad diets, including discussion of the flaws of these types of diets.

Weighing the Claims in Diet Ads

Federal Trade Commission

Web site: http://www.consumer.ftc.gov/articles/0061-weighing-claims-diet-ads

Description: Gives examples of hot topics and false claims consumers should be aware of when evaluating weight loss ads.

Weight Loss & Fitness

Federal Trade Commission

Web site: http://www.consumer.ftc.gov/topics/weight-loss-fitness

Description: Links to featured publications and facts for consumers on potential risks of dietary supplements, evaluating diet ads, and buying exercise equipment.

What You Should Know About Popular Diets

USDA, Nutrition.gov

Web site: http://www.nutrition.gov/weight-management/what-you-should-know-about-popular-diets

Description: Provides links to consumer resources on evaluating popular diets and weight loss programs.

4. Supervised Approaches to Weight Loss

DISCLAIMER:

People considering bariatric surgery (i.e., use of a band or staples to reduce the size of the stomach and/or restructuring of the digestive tract), medication, or a special diet (e.g., very low-calorie) for weight loss should first consult with a physician who can help them determine which, if any, of these methods are appropriate given their health and medical needs.

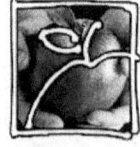

Books

The Complete Idiot's Guide to Eating Well After Weight Loss Surgery
Margaret Furtado, MS, RD, LDN, RYT and Joseph Ewing
New York: Alpha Books, 2009, 384 pp.
ISBN: 978-1592579518
Description: Discusses what to expect after surgery and proper nourishment while keeping the weight off post-surgery, and addresses challenges and how to overcome them. Also provides meal plans and recipes.

Weight Loss Surgery for Dummies, 2nd Edition
Marina Kurian, MD, FACS, Barbara Thompson, and Brian K. Davidson
Hoboken, NJ: Wiley Publishing, Inc., 2012, 384 pp.
ISBN: 1118293185
Description: Discusses who should consider weight loss surgery, types of procedures, and provides input on selecting medical centers and surgical teams to achieve a desired result. Also gives tips for preparing meals and eating well post-operatively.

Brochures, Booklets, and Tools

Weight-control Information Network
DHHS, NIH, National Institute for Diabetes and Digestive and Kidney Diseases
Web site: http://win.niddk.nih.gov/index.htm
Description: Provides the general public, health professionals, the media, and Congress with up-to-date, science-based information on weight control, obesity, physical activity, and related nutritional issues.
Ordering Information:
The Weight-control Information Network
1 WIN Way
Bethesda, MD 20892-3665
Phone: 1-877-946-4627
Fax: 202-828-1028
Publications Order Form: http://win.niddk.nih.gov/order/orderpub.htm
Email: win@info.niddk.nih.gov

Bariatric Surgery for Severe Obesity
Full text: http://win.niddk.nih.gov/publications/gastric.htm
Description: Reviews what the surgery entails, and discusses risks and benefits as well as the cost involved. Also provides additional resources.

Prescription Medications for the Treatment of Obesity
Full text: http://win.niddk.nih.gov/publications/prescription.htm
Description: Discusses uses of specific types of medications, their benefits/risks, as well as who might benefit from the use of these medications. The pamphlet ends with a frequently asked questions section.

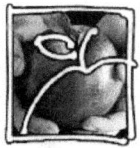

Very Low-calorie Diets
Full text: http://win.niddk.nih.gov/publications/low_calorie.htm
Description: Discusses the uses and dangers of very low calorie diets (typically, less than 800 calories per day) for weight loss.

Web Sites

Gastric Bypass Diet: What to Eat After the Surgery
MayoClinic.com, Mayo Foundation for Medical Education and Research
Web site: http://www.mayoclinic.com/health/gastric-bypass-diet/MY00827/METHOD=print
Description: Describes a diet specifically designed for people who have just had gastric bypass surgery and notes changes to eating habits to ensure safe weight loss. Risks of not following a gastric bypass diet as directed by a physician are also included.

Obesity Treatments: Bariatric Surgery
Obesity Action Coalition
Web site: http://www.obesityaction.org/obesity-treatments/bariatric-surgery
Description: Discusses types of weight-loss surgery, indications for surgery, advantages and potential complications of each one, and advises careful consultation with a doctor before deciding whether surgery is the right option.

Obesity Treatments: Physician-supervised Weight-loss
Obesity Action Coalition
Web site: http://www.obesityaction.org/obesity-treatments/physician-supervised-programs
Description: Reviews weight management options, including diet and behavior modification, medication, and referrals to related services, under the guidance of a physician.

Over-the-Counter Weight-loss Pills: Do They Work?
MayoClinic.com, Mayo Foundation for Medical Education and Research
Web site: http://www.mayoclinic.com/health/weight-loss/HQ01160/METHOD=print
Description: A review of several non-prescription weight-loss pills (including herbal or dietary supplements), and the claims, side effects, and potential pitfalls of weight-loss pills.

Weight Loss Surgery
NIH, National Library of Medicine, MedlinePlus
Web site: http://www.nlm.nih.gov/medlineplus/weightlosssurgery.html
Description: Provides a brief overview of weight loss surgery, and gives links to overviews, news, and related issues.

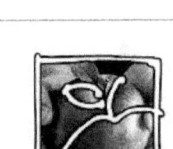

D. Weight Management Resources for Children and Adolescents

Books

Eat! Move! Play! A Parent's Guide for Raising Healthy, Happy Kids
Weight Watchers
Hoboken, NJ: John Wiley & Sons, Inc., 2010, 240 pp.
ISBN: 9780470474204
Description: Guides parents in teaching their children how to develop a positive body image, choose healthy foods (includes recipes), and exercise regularly.

Healthy Eating, Healthy Weight for Kids and Teens
Jodie Shield, MEd, RD and Mary Catherine Mullen, MS, RD
Chicago, IL: Academy of Nutrition and Dietetics, 2012, 288 pp.
ISBN: 0983725500
Description: Resource for parents that provides tips and strategies to promote a healthy weight in school age children using eight successful strategies as recommended by the Academy of Nutrition and Dietetics. Includes menus and recipes for families with children.

Keeping Kids Fit: A Family Plan for Raising Active, Healthy Children
Len Saunders
New York, NY: La Chance Publishing LLC, 2010, 225 pp.
ISBN: 1934184268
Description: Presents parents and caregivers with activity ideas and suggestions for promoting a healthy family lifestyle. It includes nutrition information and a list of exercises.

Red Light, Green Light, Eat Right
Joanna Dolgoff, MD
New York, NY: Rodale Inc., 2010, 272 pp.
ISBN: 1605294845
Description: Book for parents that uses the method of using traffic light colors to divide food into three categories – Go, Slow, and Uh Oh – to help families make healthy choices in their diet.

Brochures, Booklets, and Tools

Childhood Nutrition: Preventing Obesity
InJoy Videos, 2012
Description: This 2-volume DVD set provides parents and caregivers with information to help prevent childhood obesity starting from birth through age 5. Information is provided on breastfeeding, starting solids, selecting baby foods, promoting family meals, increasing food variety and reducing mealtime conflicts.
Ordering Information:
Phone: 800-326-2082   Fax: 303-449-8788
Web site: www.injoyvideos.com

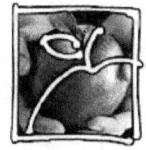

Eat Right & Move: Healthy Living for Young Families

Joanna Wiggins Garofalo

Franklin, VA: LA Publishing, 2010

Description: This booklet outlines basic tips and ideas for parents and is separated into two sections on nutrition and physical activity.

Ordering Information:

LA Publishing, LLC

P.O. Box 773

Franklin, VA 23851

Phone: 800-397-5833   Fax: 804-744-602

Email: office@breastfeedingbooks.com

Happy Mealtimes & Healthy Kids

Learning ZoneXpress, 2011

Description: In this DVD, viewers will learn that parents and children have separate roles to play in regard to eating: the parent decides what, when, and where food is served; the child decides whether or not to eat and if so, how much to eat.

Ordering Information:

Phone: 888-455-7003   Email: customersupport@learningzonexpress.com

Web site: http://www.learningzonexpress.com/

Help Me Be Healthy Series

Crabtree and Company, Inc.

Description: Offers guidance on child health and nutrition issues from birth through five years of age. Also available in Spanish.

Ordering Information:

Crabtree and Company, Inc.

200 Park Avenue

Falls Church, VA 22046

Phone: 888-531-9001 ext. 102

Email: info@helpmebehealthy.net

Online ordering: http://helpmebehealthy.net/order.html

Helping Your Child: Tips for Parents

DHHS, NIH, NIDDK, Weight-control Information Network

Full text: http://win.niddk.nih.gov/publications/child.htm

Description: Highlights ways parents can encourage healthy eating and physical activity within their families.

Ordering Information:

The Weight-control Information Network

1 WIN Way

Bethesda, MD 20892-3665

Phone: 1-877-946-4627   Fax: 202-828-1028

Publications Order Form: http://win.niddk.nih.gov/order/orderpub.htm

Email: win@info.niddk.nih.gov

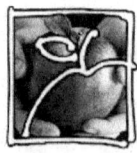

Your Child's Healthy Weight
Channing Bete Company Inc., 2011
Description: This booklet provides ways to help a child develop healthy eating habits, shape a child's attitude toward food and exercise. It discusses how to tell if a child is overweight and how being overweight can impact children's physical and emotional health.
Ordering Information:
Phone: 800-477-4776   Email: custsvcs@channing-bete.com
Web site: www.channing-bete.com/

Web Sites

Alliance for a Healthier Generation
American Heart Association; William J. Clinton Foundation
Web site: http://www.healthiergeneration.org
Description: Works to reduce childhood obesity by 2015 and encourage kids to make healthy choices. Provides resources for teachers, parents, and healthcare providers to help kids eat healthier and move more.

BMI Percentile Calculator for Child and Teen
DHHS, Centers for Disease Control and Prevention
Web site: http://apps.nccd.cdc.gov/dnpabmi/Calculator.aspx
Description: Calculates body mass index (BMI) for children and teens ages 2-19 years. Information on interpreting BMI values can be found on a corresponding Web page, "About BMI for Children and Teens," located here:
http://www.cdc.gov/healthyweight/assessing/bmi/childrens_BMI/about_childrens_BMI.html

Childhood Obesity Facts
DHHS, Centers for Disease Control and Prevention
Web site: http://cdc.gov/healthyyouth/obesity/
Description: Provides data and statistics, along with links to science-based strategies that schools and communities can use to combat childhood obesity.

Childhood Overweight
Obesity Society
Web site: http://www.obesity.org/resources-for/childhood-overweight.htm
Description: Provides prevalence of childhood obesity as well as tips to help parents and caregivers establish healthy eating patterns with kids.

A Healthy Weight
DHHS, Office on Women's Health
Web site: http://girlshealth.gov/nutrition/healthyweight/index.cfm
Description: Advice for girls ages 10 to 16 on how to achieve a healthy weight.

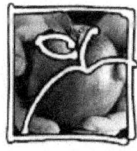

Is Dieting OK for Kids?
Nemours Foundation
Full text:
http://kidshealth.org/PageManager.jsp?dn=KidsHealth&lic=1&ps=307&cat_id=119&article_set=22521
Description: Discusses why dieting may be inappropriate for children and provides suggestions for things kids can do to stay at a healthy weight.

Let's Move!
The White House; USDA; DHHS; Department of Education; Department of the Interior
Web site: http://www.letsmove.gov
Description: Supports First Lady Michelle Obama's comprehensive initiative dedicated to solving the problem of obesity within a generation. Provides access to resources on healthy eating, getting active, taking action and joining the movement.

MyPlate for Preschoolers and Children Over Five
USDA, Center for Nutrition Policy and Promotion
- **MyPlate for Preschoolers**
  Web site: http://www.choosemyplate.gov/preschoolers.html
  Description: Encourages healthy eating and physical activity behaviors for children ages 2-5. Includes sections on growth, dealing with a picky eater, and food safety.
- **MyPlate for Children Over Five**
  Web site: http://www.choosemyplate.gov/children-over-five.html
  Description: Designed to motivate children ages 6-11 to make healthy food choices and be physically active. The Web site includes worksheets, an online game and tips for parents.

Nourish Interactive
Nourish Interactive
Web site: http://www.nourishinteractive.com/
Description: Includes online games, blogs, health-hint calendars, and newsletters for kids as well as lesson plans and worksheets for parents.

Obesity: Healthychildren.org
American Academy of Pediatrics
Web site: http://www.healthychildren.org/English/health-issues/conditions/obesity/Pages/default.aspx
Description: Provides various articles and resources on childhood obesity and its prevention among children and teens, and offers assessment and evaluation worksheets (e.g., assessing your home environment and evaluating snacking behaviors) for parents.

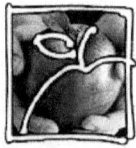

Obesity in Children
Obesity Action Coalition
Web site: http://www.obesityaction.org/understanding-obesity-in-children
Description: Defines childhood obesity and explains potential causes of childhood obesity. Also discusses appropriate measures of weight for children, addresses the stigma of childhood obesity, and provides kid-friendly resources in the "Kid's Corner."

Obesity in Children
NIH, National Library of Medicine, MedlinePlus
Web site: http://www.nlm.nih.gov/medlineplus/obesityinchildren.html
Description: Provides an overview of obesity in children and links to helpful resources on news, treatment and prevention.

Reducing Childhood Obesity
Academy of Nutrition and Dietetics
Web site: http://www.eatright.org/childhoodobesity/
Description: Resources for parents and care-givers to teach children about healthy foods, practice what they teach and make sure physical activity is incorporated into each day.

Tips for Parents – Ideas to Help Children Maintain a Healthy Weight
DHHS, Centers for Disease Control and Prevention
Web site: http://www.cdc.gov/healthyweight/children/index.html
Description: Addresses concerns related to the risks of childhood obesity and provides tips on how parents can help prevent it.

We Can! Ways to Enhance Children's Activity & Nutrition
DHHS, NIH, National Heart Lung and Blood Institute
Web site: http://www.nhlbi.nih.gov/health/public/heart/obesity/wecan/
Description: Supports families and communities in helping children maintain a healthy weight. The program focuses on improving food choices, increasing physical activity and reducing screen time. Spanish materials also available here:
http://www.nhlbi.nih.gov/health/public/heart/obesity/wecan/espanol/index.htm.

This resource list was updated and compiled by:
Kathleen Pellechia, RD, Nutrition Information Specialist
Sara Wilson, MS, RD, Nutrition Information Specialist

Acknowledgment is given to the following FNIC reviewers:
Jennifer Mitchell, BA, Nutrition Information Assistant
Shirley King Evans, EdM, RD, Budget Analyst

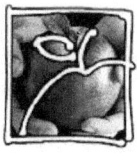

This publication was developed in part through a Cooperative Agreement with the Department of Nutrition and Food Science in the College of Agriculture and Natural Resources at the University of Maryland.

Locate additional FNIC publications at http://fnic.nal.usda.gov/resourcelists.

Food and Nutrition Information Center
Agricultural Research Service, USDA
National Agricultural Library, Room 108
10301 Baltimore Avenue
Beltsville, MD 20705-2351
Phone: 301-504-5414
Fax: 301-504-6409
TTY: 301-504-6856
Contact: http://fnic.nal.usda.gov/contact
Web site: http://fnic.nal.usda.gov

The National Agricultural Library (NAL) provides lending and photocopying services to U.S. Department of Agriculture (USDA) employees. Non-USDA users can obtain materials from NAL through the interlibrary lending services of their local, corporate, or university library. For further information on NAL's document delivery services visit their Web site at http://www.nal.usda.gov/nal-services/request-library-materials.

For questions on document delivery services please call 301-504-5717 or submit a question at http://www.nal.usda.gov/ask-question-3.

The use of trade, firm, or corporation names in this publication (or page) is for the information and convenience of the reader. Such use does not constitute an official endorsement or approval by the USDA or the Agricultural Research Service (ARS) of any product or service to the exclusion of others that may be suitable.

USDA prohibits discrimination in all its programs and activities on the basis of race, color, national origin, age, disability, and where applicable, sex, marital status, familial status, parental status, religion, sexual orientation, genetic information, political beliefs, reprisal, or because all or a part of an individual's income is derived from any public assistance program. (Not all prohibited bases apply to all programs.)

Persons with disabilities who require alternative means for communication of program information (Braille, large print, audiotape, etc.) should contact USDA's TARGET Center at 202-720-2600 (voice and TDD).

To file a complaint of discrimination write to USDA, Director, Office of Adjudication, 1400 Independence Avenue, S.W., Washington, D.C. 20250-9410 or call 800-632-9992 (voice) or 202-401-0216 (TDD). USDA is an equal opportunity provider and employer.

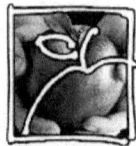